Aspir

A manual guide that teach about nonsteroidal anti-inflammatory drug used to relieve mild to moderate pain, lower fever and lower the risk of serious problems like strokes and heart attacks

Dr. Tyler K. Kevin

Table of Contents

Chapter One

Introduction to Aspirin

The classic nonsteroidal anti-inflammatory medicine (NSAID) aspirin has been used for a variety of ailments and has stood the test of time. For more than a century, people have kept this medication, also known as acetylsalicylic acid, in their medicine cabinets. When its pain-relieving abilities were initially identified in the late 19th century, its extraordinary adventure began. It has since evolved into a pillar in the treatment of inflammation, fever, and pain.

The primary benefits of aspirin are its effectiveness in decreasing fever and relieving mild to moderate discomfort. Its effects range widely, from small injuries and rheumatic stiffness to headaches and tooth pain. The significance of aspirin goes beyond these immediate effects to include its part in cardiovascular health. Aspirin is a crucial part of preventive cardiology since it has a critical function in lowering the risk of heart attacks and strokes through its capacity to inhibit blood clot formation.

Aspirin interferes with the formation of prostaglandins, which is the mechanism of action behind its therapeutic effects. Chemical messengers known as prostaglandins are a factor in heat, discomfort, and inflammation. Aspirin decreases inflammation and relieves pain by preventing the formation of these substances. Additionally, it has significant effects on cardiovascular health by avoiding the formation of clots that could cause serious health issues. This is because it can suppress platelet aggregation.

Thoughts and intricacies are not unimportant when using aspirin. It provides a number of advantages, but there are also potential drawbacks and hazards, which emphasizes the significance of using it responsibly. The effectiveness of aspirin as a medicine depends on a number of variables, including dosage, frequency of use, and personal health state. To guarantee safe and efficient use, it's essential to speak with a doctor before starting an Aspirin regimen.

Chapter Two

Aspirin Uses for Pain Relief

An effective remedy for a variety of discomforts is aspirin, a mainstay in the field of pain management. Because of its capacity to alter how the body interprets pain signals, it is effective at reducing pain. Aspirin accomplishes this by preventing the synthesis of prostaglandins, which are the molecules that send signals to the brain related to pain and inflammation. Aspirin lessens the severity of pain sensations and provides comfort by preventing the production of prostaglandins.

Aspirin has established itself as a flexible analgesic, providing relief from a variety of pains, including the typical headache, muscular pain, and even the discomfort related to dental treatments. It is an excellent alternative for people looking for relief from minor to moderate aches and pains because of its effectiveness in treating mild to moderate pain. People can now manage minor pain without the need for ongoing medical monitoring because to its non-prescription availability.

Aspirin is also useful for illnesses where pain is brought on by inflammation due to its anti-inflammatory effects. Aspirin has a dual effect that relieves pain while also reducing inflammation, which is beneficial for conditions like arthritis where joint inflammation causes discomfort. By targeting both the underlying inflammatory processes and the sensory experience of pain, its holistic approach differentiates it as a complete solution for pain management.

The use of aspirin should follow established dosages and recommendations even though it can be an efficient painkiller. For those with pre-existing medical disorders or those using other medications, it is best to speak with a healthcare provider before adding aspirin to a pain management regimen. Aspirin can be a helpful tool in the search of pain relief and enhanced quality of life when used sensibly, with knowledge, and after considering all available options.

Aspirin Uses in Lowering Fever

A dependable ally in the fight to lower fever is aspirin, which is well known for its wide range of medicinal uses. The body attempts to overcome these problems by raising its internal temperature, which leads to fever, which is frequently a sign of an underlying illness or inflammation. The ability of aspirin to influence the production of prostaglandins, which is crucial for both starting and maintaining the body's fever response, is a critical factor in its ability to reduce fever.

Aspirin successfully reduces the body's capacity to produce a fever by interfering with the production of prostaglandins. As a result, it can serve as an antipyretic and assist in lowering high body temperatures to more tolerable levels. Aspirin's effect on fever is most notable in situations of viral or bacterial infections, where reducing fever not only relieves discomfort but also enhances the body's immunological response by fostering an environment that is more favorable for immune cells to respond to stimuli effectively.

It is important to remember that even while aspirin can be useful in lowering fever, its use should be cautious. For people with particular medical conditions or those who are on other drugs, it is extremely important to follow the suggested dosages and seek medical advice. Aspirin's function in lowering fever is just one aspect of how it is used more generally to promote comfort and wellbeing, enhancing its reputation as a flexible instrument in the world of medical interventions.

It's crucial to note that Reye's syndrome, a rare but deadly disorder that damages the liver and brain, should be avoided in some circumstances, especially among children and teenagers, and that Aspirin should only be administered under close supervision. Since this age group may benefit from other fever-reducing strategies, healthcare practitioners may suggest them. To use aspirin's fever-reducing advantages safely and efficiently, responsible usage and well-informed choices are necessary in every situation.

Aspirin Uses for Blood Thinning and Cardiovascular Health

Beyond reducing pain and fever, aspirin is important because of its vital role in supporting cardiovascular health because to its blood-thinning effects. Inhibiting platelet aggregation, a crucial step in the creation of blood clots, is one of its most noteworthy applications. Aspirin aids in preventing the growth of potentially fatal blood clots that could obstruct vital arteries and result in heart attacks or strokes by reducing the clumping together of platelets.

Aspirin has become a staple in preventive cardiology because of this special quality. Under the direction of medical specialists, low-dose aspirin may be recommended to those who are susceptible to cardiovascular events, such as those who have a history of heart disease or stroke. This application aims to reduce the chance of clot development and preserve blood flow to essential organs. Aspirin's blood-thinning action may also be used to avoid clots and hasten recovery after some cardiovascular procedures, like the implantation of stents.

It's crucial to understand that while aspirin's blood-thinning effects are advantageous, they should be used with care. Individual risk factors and medical advice should be considered when deciding whether to use aspirin for cardiovascular health. The advantages must be balanced against possible concerns, such as heightened bleeding susceptibility. To establish a balanced strategy that maximizes cardiovascular protection without compromising general wellbeing, responsible usage and adherence to authorized dosages are essential.

Beyond its acute blood-thinning effects, aspirin has long-term effects on cardiovascular health. According to studies, long-term, low-dose aspirin use may provide anti-inflammatory advantages that support its cardio protective effects. However, continuing research is helping to clarify our knowledge of aspirin's complex role in cardiovascular health and direct the most efficient and secure way to use it. Aspirin's continued importance in the effort to preserve a healthy heart and circulatory system is underlined by its capacity to improve blood flow, lower the risk of clotting, and maybe provide anti-inflammatory properties.

Chapter Three

Mechanism of Action

Blocking the Synthesis of Prostaglandins

Aspirin's complex mechanism of action, particularly its function in preventing the production of prostaglandins, is at the core of its potency. Prostaglandins are hormone-like substances that act as signaling molecules within the body and are essential for a number of physiological functions, such as inflammation, pain perception, and temperature regulation. Cyclooxygenases (COX), which are released by cells in response to tissue damage or inflammation, help to produce prostaglandins. Prostaglandins in turn enhance pain signals and cause inflammatory reactions.

Aspirin has the ability to acetylate substances, which causes an irreversible inhibition of COX enzyme activity. It focuses more particularly on a certain COX-1 form of the enzyme. This COX activity blockade stops the synthesis of prostaglandins, effectively decreasing inflammation and lowering pain signals. Due to its powerful analgesic and anti-inflammatory properties, aspirin is used to treat a variety of pain-related ailments, from small aches to long-term inflammatory diseases like arthritis.

Preventing Platelet Aggregation

Aspirin has significant effects on prostaglandins in addition to its ability to prevent platelet aggregation, which is very important when considering cardiovascular health. Blood cells called platelets are crucial in the process of clot formation, which helps to control bleeding when wounds are sustained. The creation of clots that obstruct blood flow and can cause serious cardiovascular events like heart attacks and strokes is however possible when platelets cluster excessively within blood arteries.

By permanently suppressing the cyclooxygenase-1 (COX-1) enzyme found in platelets, aspirin interferes with this process. The enzyme COX-1 is essential for the synthesis of thromboxane A2, which encourages platelet aggregation and vasoconstriction. Aspirin reduces platelet aggregation and inhibits the formation of blood clots via inhibiting COX-1, which in turn decreases the creation of thromboxane A2.

Because of its antithrombotic properties, aspirin is now a crucial aspect of cardiovascular therapy, especially for those who are at high risk of cardiovascular events. Low-dose aspirin may be recommended as a preventative measure for people with a history of heart disease or stroke. When using aspirin to manage cardiovascular health, it is crucial to carefully weigh the benefits of blood thinning against the risk of bleeding issues. This highlights the significance of receiving personalized medical guidance.

In conclusion, aspirin's twin modes of action—inhibiting both prostaglandin synthesis and platelet aggregation—emphasize its adaptability in treating pain, inflammation, and cardiovascular health. Aspirin has changed the landscape of medical interventions by focusing on fundamental processes at the molecular level and providing protection and alleviation for a variety of medical disorders.

Chapter Four

Recommended Dosages of Aspirin for Different Conditions

Depending on the intended purpose and the patient's health, different aspirin dosages are recommended. Before adding aspirin to your regular medication regimen, it's critical to adhere to suggested dosages and seek medical advice. The general recommendations for aspirin doses for various illnesses are provided below:

Pain Relief and Fever Reduction: The recommended dosage of aspirin for people seeking pain relief or fever reduction is 325 to 650 milligrams (mg), administered orally as needed every 4 to 6 hours. A daily dose of aspirin should not exceed 4 grams (4000 mg). It may be necessary to adjust the dosage based on the severity of the discomfort or temperature as well as the patient's response. Children and teens under the age of 18 should refrain from taking aspirin for fever because they run the risk of contracting Reye's syndrome, a rare but fatal condition.

Cardiovascular Health: lessen doses of aspirin are frequently advised for people using it to lessen their risk of cardiovascular events. A low-dose aspirin regimen typically consists of 81 milligrams (mg) administered once daily. This dosage effectively prevents platelet aggregation and lowers the risk of blood clot formation without raising the risk of consequences from bleeding. However, the choice to use aspirin for cardiovascular health should be made in cooperation with a healthcare professional, taking into consideration personal health history and risk factors.

Higher doses of aspirin may be necessary when treating chronic inflammatory disorders like arthritis. The suggested dosage can differ, but a typical range is 2 to 4 grams (2000 to 4000 mg) each day, divided into many doses. When using aspirin for extended periods of time at larger dosages, it's critical to work closely with a healthcare provider to watch for any potential side effects and interactions.

Preventive Use in precise Situations: In some cases, such as before particular medical procedures or surgeries, healthcare professionals may recommend a brief course of aspirin at precise dosages to avoid blood clot development. The dosage will be decided based on the patient's health, the procedure being done, and the desired amount of anti-platelet action.

Always put responsible use first by sticking to the recommended dosages and avoiding changing the dosage without seeing a doctor. Additionally, to be sure there are no possible interactions, let your healthcare professional know about any additional medications you are taking. While aspirin has a number of advantages, using it safely and effectively requires making well-informed decisions and working together with a healthcare provider.

Aspirin Administration Guidelines

To maximize the effectiveness of aspirin and reduce the danger of side effects, aspirin must be administered properly. A safe and beneficial experience is made more likely by following the directions for taking aspirin. Here are some essential administrative guidelines to bear in mind:

Follow the dosage recommendations supplied by your healthcare provider or listed on the prescription label. Take the recommended dosage with a full glass of water to promote absorption and reduce the possibility of stomach lining discomfort. Depending on the aspirin dosage's intended use, different times may be required for delivery. It is typically advised to take aspirin every 4 to 6 hours as needed for pain relief or fever decrease. A low-dose plan may comprise taking Aspirin once per day for cardiovascular health.

Consider taking aspirin with food or a glass of milk to lessen the possibility of stomach irritation or discomfort. This can lessen the possibility of gastrointestinal adverse effects and assist in forming a protective barrier in the stomach. Additionally, before beginning aspirin therapy, speak with your doctor to identify the best way of administration if you have a history of stomach ulcers or gastrointestinal problems.

Avoid Crushing or Chewing: Unless specifically told to do so by your healthcare professional, it's crucial to swallow the aspirin tablet whole and not to crush, break, or chew it. Its intended release mechanism may be altered and its absorption may be impacted by breaking the pill.

Compliance and Consistency: If you're using aspirin as part of a preventive program for cardiovascular health, try to be consistent with how often you take it. A medication's advantages may be diminished by missed doses or inconsistent use. Establish a regular schedule to take Aspirin to help with compliance.

Consult your healthcare professional before beginning an aspirin regimen, especially if you have any pre-existing problems, are taking any other medications, are pregnant, or are nursing. Based on the specifics of your health profile, they can offer you individualized advice on the right dosage, timing, and safety measures.

Potential Interactions: Be wary of any interactions with additional prescription drugs or dietary supplements you may be taking. Nonsteroidal anti-inflammatory drugs (NSAIDs) or certain blood thinners may interact with aspirin and reduce or increase the effectiveness of the drug or the risk of bleeding.

To summarize, following the aspirin administration instructions is essential for maximizing its advantages while lowering any possible hazards. It is possible to have a safe and effective experience with this drug by working with a healthcare provider, being consistent with your dosage, and using the suggested precautions.

Aspirin Safety Precautions and Unique Considerations

Despite the fact that aspirin has a wide variety of advantages, it is crucial to be aware of the precautions and unique considerations to ensure its safe and efficient usage. Making educated decisions and avoiding potential pitfalls both benefit from your understanding of these factors. Observe the following important details:

A history of allergies to nonsteroidal anti-inflammatory medicines (NSAIDs) or any other medications should be disclosed to your healthcare professional before taking aspirin. An allergic reaction to aspirin may present as hives, rash, breathing problems, or swelling, and such reactions call for emergency medical intervention.

Health of the Gastrointestinal Tract: Aspirin can aggravate the stomach lining and may be a factor in the development of gastrointestinal ulcers or bleeding, particularly when used frequently or in larger dosages. Before beginning treatment, patients with a history of gastrointestinal problems, bleeding disorders, or stomach ulcers should talk to their doctor about the advantages and disadvantages of using aspirin. Aspirin can lessen gastrointestinal discomfort when used with food or milk.

Bleeding Risks: Prior to surgery or dental operations, it's crucial to take into account how aspirin's blood-thinning effects may raise the risk of bleeding. Your healthcare practitioner may advise interim Aspirin withdrawal or dosage change to reduce bleeding risks, so it's critical to let them know about any planned surgeries or dental procedures.

Drug Interactions: Aspirin may interact with other medications, such as NSAIDs, anticoagulants, blood thinners, and herbal supplements, to magnify its effects or raise the risk of bleeding. To enable them to look for potential interactions and modify your treatment plan as necessary, always provide your healthcare provider a thorough list of all the drugs and supplements you are taking.

Breastfeeding: Using aspirin when breastfeeding or pregnant calls for careful caution. If you are pregnant, intend to become pregnant, or are breast-feeding, speak with your healthcare professional before using aspirin. It's vital to heed medical advice because using aspirin in high doses or for an extended period of time while pregnant could cause difficulties.

Children and teenagers: Due to the possibility of developing Reye's syndrome, an uncommon but deadly illness that affects the brain and liver, aspirin use in children and teenagers is generally discouraged. For this age group, alternatives like ibuprofen or acetaminophen are frequently suggested.

Chronic Health disorders: Before taking aspirin, people with chronic health disorders such asthma, renal illness, liver disease, or a history of stroke should talk to their doctor. Aspirin use may necessitate close observation and possible dosage modifications.

In conclusion, while aspirin has many advantages, using it responsibly requires being alert and cautious. You may jointly decide the safest and most efficient method for utilizing aspirin for your health needs by being open and honest with your healthcare practitioner about your medical history, current illnesses, and any drugs you are taking. You may take advantage of Aspirin's benefits while limiting dangers by prioritizing appropriate usage and adhering to medical advice.

Chapter Five

Potential Aspirin Benefits and Risks

Aspirin has a variety of possible advantages, including the ability to relieve pain, lower fevers, and promote cardiovascular health. It does, however, have some hazards, just like any prescription, which must be evaluated against the benefits. Making wise choices regarding the use of aspirin requires a thorough understanding of both its possible advantages and hazards.

Benefits:

Aspirin is an effective analgesic for treating mild to moderate pain and lowering fever because it can suppress the production of prostaglandins. Its numerous uses include treating dental discomfort as well as menstrual cramps and headaches, as well as muscular and joint pain. Aspirin serves as a common over-the-counter pain medication due to its efficiency in stifling pain signals and lowering inflammation.

Cardiovascular Protection: The ability of aspirin to reduce the risk of cardiovascular events is one of its most noteworthy advantages. Aspirin has a crucial role in lowering the risk of heart attacks and strokes by decreasing platelet aggregation and blood clot formation. For people with a history of heart disease or those who are vulnerable to difficulties from blood clots, this cardiovascular protection is especially beneficial.

Aspirin's anti-inflammatory properties make it a useful tool in the treatment of diseases like arthritis that are characterized by inflammation. It helps to lessen swelling and discomfort related to inflammatory illnesses by reducing the formation of prostaglandins.

Risks:

Gastrointestinal Irritation: The effects of aspirin on the stomach lining may cause gastrointestinal irritation, which may eventually result in ulcers or bleeding, particularly with long-term or high-dose use. People who have a history of digestive problems like ulcers or bleeding disorders are more susceptible and should use cautious or look into alternate therapies.

Risks of Bleeding: Aspirin's blood-thinning effects can raise the risk of bleeding, which is especially important prior to surgeries, dental treatments, or when combined with other blood-thinning drugs. Before using aspirin, patients should talk to their doctor if they have a bleeding disorder or are taking an anticoagulant.

Allergic responses: Although uncommon, aspirin can cause allergic responses, which can show up as hives, rash, breathing problems, or swelling. People who have a history of allergies to NSAIDs or other drugs must to be cautious and get medical help right once if any adverse symptoms appear.

Risk-Benefit Evaluation

It is important to carefully weigh the potential advantages and disadvantages of aspirin. The evaluation of a person's medical history, current health issues, and potential drug interactions by healthcare providers is crucial. The choice to use aspirin should be made in conjunction with the individual's health and safety, with a focus on tailored treatment strategies.

In conclusion, aspirin has long been known to be effective for treating pain, lowering fever, and protecting the cardiovascular system. Its hazards, such as gastrointestinal distress, a propensity for bleeding, and potential allergic reactions, must be understood, though. Individuals can modify their use of aspirin to optimize benefits while limiting hazards by consulting with a healthcare professional before making any decisions.

Aspirin Interactions with Other Medications

To ensure your safety and the efficacy of your treatment plan, it is essential to understand any possible interactions between aspirin and other medications. Aspirin's special abilities as an anti-inflammatory and blood thinner may affect how it interacts with other medications. Here are factors to remember:

Blood-Thinning Drugs: Combining aspirin with other blood-thinning drugs, such as anticoagulants (warfarin, heparin) or antiplatelet medicines (clopidogrel, ticagrelor), can increase the risk of bleeding. Combining these two substances may increase the blood-thinning effect and increase the risk of life-threatening bleeding problems. Healthcare professionals carefully weigh the advantages and disadvantages of combining these drugs, frequently modifying dosages to strike the right balance between lowering the risk of bleeding and maintaining therapeutic benefits.

Nonsteroidal Anti-Inflammatory Drugs (NSAIDs): Combining aspirin with other NSAIDs (ibuprofen, naproxen) can lessen aspirin's tendency to thin the blood. This is brought on by competition for the same enzymes involved in the antiplatelet action. Before taking any other NSAIDs, it's crucial to talk to your doctor if you have been prescribed low-dose aspirin for cardiovascular protection. They may suggest different painkillers to avoid interfering with aspirin's beneficial effects.

When combined with aspirin, long-term usage of corticosteroids like prednisone can raise the risk of gastrointestinal bleeding. Healthcare professionals might advise taking precautions to lessen this risk, like taking a stomach protectant or lowering the dosage of one or both medications.

Antacids and stomach acid reducers: Some antacids or stomach acid reducers (proton pump inhibitors, H2 blockers) can affect how well aspirin is absorbed and may lessen its effectiveness. Talk to your doctor about how these medications may affect the effects of aspirin if you take them for stomach problems.

Aspirin may potentially interact with herbal supplements and over-the-counter medicines. For instance, ginkgo biloba, ginger, and garlic might intensify the blood-thinning effects of aspirin, raising the risk of bleeding. To make sure they are compatible with your Aspirin regimen, you should always let your healthcare provider know about any supplements or over-the-counter drugs you are taking.

Consult Your Healthcare Professional: Openly discuss your entire pharmaceutical regimen with your doctor when you are prescribed aspirin or considering using it. They will take into account probable interactions and advise you on how to modify dosages, treatment regimens, or pick different medications if necessary. You can maximize the safety and effectiveness of your treatment while lowering the risks connected with the use of many medications by proactively addressing potential interactions.

Chapter Six

Frequently Asked Questions about Aspirin

1. Is it okay to take aspirin before food?

Yes, you can take aspirin on an empty stomach. To lessen the possibility of stomach irritation or pain, take it with food or a glass of milk. Consult your healthcare professional for advice on modifying administration techniques if you encounter any digestive problems while taking aspirin.

2. Is long-term usage of aspirin safe?

Low-dose aspirin is generally safe to use for a prolonged period of time, especially when used in accordance with medical advice. The decision to use aspirin for a prolonged period of time should be based on your medical history, risk factors, and any potential drug interactions. Your health can be monitored and the treatment plan can be changed as needed with regular check-ups with your healthcare practitioner.

3. Can I use aspirin when nursing or pregnant?

Before using aspirin, it's vital to talk to your doctor if you are breastfeeding, trying to get pregnant, or already pregnant. Complications could arise from the prolonged or high-dose use of aspirin during pregnancy. Your healthcare professional will assist you in balancing the risks and advantages of using aspirin and give advice regarding whether it is right for you.

4. Can youngsters and children take aspirin for a fever?

Due to the possibility of Reye's syndrome, a rare but deadly disorder that damages the liver and brain, it is typically advised against providing aspirin to children and teenagers for fever reduction. For fever in this age group, acetaminophen or ibuprofen are frequently suggested alternatives.

5. Can I use aspirin along with other drugs?

Aspirin may interact with NSAIDs, blood thinners, herbal supplements, and other medications. For safe and efficient use, make sure to tell your healthcare professional about all of the medications and supplements you are taking. Your treatment plan will be modified as necessary by your healthcare professional after considering any potential interactions.

6. Does aspirin work to ward off heart attacks and strokes?

Low-dose As a preventative precaution, aspirin is frequently administered to people at risk for heart attacks or strokes. These cardiovascular events can be prevented by its blood-thinning effects, which prevent platelet aggregation and lower the danger of blood clots. However, the choice to use aspirin for this purpose should be based on individual risk factors and should be decided in cooperation with a healthcare professional.

7. How soon can I stop taking aspirin?

It's crucial not to abruptly cease taking aspirin without first consulting your healthcare professional if you're using it as part of a long-term treatment plan. Aspirin's effectiveness can be impacted by abrupt stopping, and there is a chance that rebound symptoms could occur. If you're thinking of quitting aspirin, talk to your doctor first to guarantee a secure and smooth transition.

8. Can aspirin trigger skin rashes or allergies?

Although uncommon, some people may experience allergic reactions or skin sensitivities to aspirin. Hives, redness, breathing problems, and swelling are just a few possible symptoms. Seek emergency medical assistance if you develop any allergy symptoms after taking aspirin.

9. I'm taking aspirin; can I drink alcohol?

The prevailing consensus is that drinking moderate amounts of alcohol while taking aspirin is safe. However, drinking too much alcohol can make you more likely to experience gastrointestinal bleeding, especially if you also take aspirin. Discuss your worries with your healthcare physician if you have any concerning alcohol use.

10. Will taking aspirin impact my ability to drive or operate equipment?

It is not known if aspirin by itself significantly impairs motor or cognitive abilities. However, it's crucial to avoid tasks that call for complete concentration until you know how Aspirin affects you if you experience dizziness, sleepiness, or any other negative effects when taking it.

11. Can I combine aspirin with over-the-counter medications?

Aspirin and other NSAIDs may be found in over-the-counter drugs like cold and pain remedies. Due to the possibility of unintended double dose, use caution while combining these products. Before combining different prescriptions, thoroughly read the medicine labels and talk to your doctor.

12. Do stomach ulcers result from aspirin use?

With extended or high-dose use, aspirin's effect on the stomach lining may make stomach irritability, ulcers, or bleeding more likely. Discuss the advantages and disadvantages of using aspirin with your healthcare physician if you have a history of stomach ulcers or gastrointestinal problems.

13. Can I take aspirin before a procedure like a dental procedure?

Tell your healthcare practitioner if you plan to use aspirin before any scheduled surgery or dental procedures. To reduce the risk of bleeding before and after the surgery, your healthcare professional can advise interim Aspirin withdrawal or dosage modifications.

14. How should I keep aspirin?

Away from dampness and bright sunlight, keep aspirin in a container at room temperature. Keep it away from pets and children. Observe the storage guidelines listed on the drug packaging.

Printed in Great Britain
by Amazon

41461680R00030